PROSTATE BIOPSY RECOVERY DIET

Transformative Nutrition Strategies And Optimize Healing For Reducing Pain And Regaining Strength

DR LUCAS KAYCE

DISCLAIMER

This book about illness and nutrition is not meant to replace expert medical advice, diagnosis, or treatment; rather, it is meant purely for informational reasons. This book's content is founded on broad concepts and recommendations for managing diseases and nutrition.

Before adopting any major dietary or lifestyle changes, readers are recommended to speak with a qualified healthcare provider, such as a licensed physician or registered dietitian, especially if they have pre-existing medical concerns. Everybody has different health demands, so what works for one person might not work for another.

The use of the information provided in this book may have unfavorable repercussions or consequences, for which the author and publisher disclaim all liability. No disease is meant to be identified, treated, cured, or prevented by the information provided.

The book may include contain references to medical literature or research findings; however readers are urged to independently confirm this material and contact reliable sources.

It is important to remember that the fields of nutrition and medicine are always changing, and that new findings could have an impact on the advice offered in this book. As a result, readers are urged to keep up with the most recent advancements in healthcare and, when in doubt, seek professional counsel.

By reading this book, readers agree that they are in charge of their own health decisions and release the author and publisher from any liability arising from the use of the material in the book, whether direct or indirect.

TABLE OF CONTENTS

ABOUT THE BOOK

The importance of diet in the healing process following a prostate biopsy is a crucial topic of healthcare that is frequently overlooked, but is covered in the book "Prostate Biopsy Recovery Diet". The need for a focused recovery diet is frequently disregarded in the field of medical literature; this book closes that gap by offering thorough instruction on the topic.

The book set the stage by explaining the details of a prostate biopsy, why it is done, and what to expect both before and after the treatment. For readers to understand the background and rationale for the need for a customized recovery diet, they must have this fundamental understanding.

The book's main focus is on nutrition throughout the healing phase, and this is emphasized. These chapters fill in the gaps between medical procedures and dietary practices by going into detail about the role nutrition plays in healing, the advantages of a Prostate Biopsy

Recovery Diet, and the unique nutritional requirements during recovery.

Readers will find helpful advice on creating a recovery diet. To help readers on their path to recovery, this book offers practical advice on everything from working with medical professionals to adjusting diets to meet specific needs and balancing minerals.

With an emphasis on details, the book lists items to consume and stay away from while recovering, along with information on anti-inflammatory choices, nutrient-dense foods, and hydration techniques. Sample meal plans are included to help readers put theory into practice even more.

The book covers long-term nutritional plans, lifestyle factors, and the function of supplements in addition to food guidance. Recipes specifically designed for prostate biopsy recovery are included in the book to give readers a complete toolkit to aid in their recovery.

For those navigating the healing process following a prostate biopsy, this book is an invaluable resource due to its insightful and well-structured information. It gives them the information and useful tools they need to maximize their dietary intake, which eventually makes the healing process go more smoothly and successfully.

CHAPTER ONE

PROSTATE BIOPSY RECOVERY DIET OVERVIEW

THE SIGNIFICANCE OF A DIET FOR PROSTATE BIOPSY RECOVERY

It is impossible to overestimate the significance of a Prostate Biopsy Recovery Diet because it is essential for speeding up the healing process and reducing pain for those who have had a prostate biopsy. A diet high in nutrients and well-balanced can help control any negative effects and greatly aid in the general healing process. Given the sensitivity of the prostate gland and the possible effects of the biopsy process on the body, this nutritional emphasis is especially important.

COMPREHENDING PROSTATE BIOPSY

Comprehending Prostate Biopsy is crucial for anyone handling this medical process. Samples of tissue from the prostate gland are removed during a prostate biopsy to look for anomalies or potential cancerous growths.

When additional diagnostic testing, including blood tests or imaging scans, points to possible problems, the operation is frequently advised. The outcomes of a prostate biopsy are crucial in choosing the right treatment plan and overseeing the patient's general health.

PROSTATE BIOPSY OVERVIEW

A synopsis of prostate biopsy highlights the importance of this procedure in the fields of cancer and urology. This diagnostic process plays a critical role in the timely identification of prostate cancer, a common and possibly fatal disorder that affects men.

To have a thorough understanding of the biopsy procedure, one must be aware of the different procedures used, such as transperineal biopsy or transrectal ultrasound-guided biopsy. The particulars of each situation must be taken into consideration, as well as the medical professional's judgment.

CAUSES OF PROSTATE BIOPSIES

Prostate biopsies are usually performed because previous tests have suggested possible problems, and a clear diagnosis is needed. Early identification of prostate cancer is typically difficult because the disease frequently exhibits unclear signs. For clinicians to precisely determine the existence and severity of prostate cancer, a biopsy becomes an essential tool. Additional justifications for a prostate biopsy could be tracking the advancement of established ailments, examining high PSA levels, or assessing anomalies found throughout a physical examination.

WHAT TO ANTICIPATE BOTH DURING AND FOLLOWING THE SURGERY

An important thing for anyone getting a prostate biopsy is to know what to anticipate both during and after the surgery. To obtain tissue samples, a tiny needle is inserted into the prostate gland during the actual surgery. Although generally regarded as safe, people may feel some minor discomfort or transient side effects like bleeding, infection, or urological problems. Essential elements include post-biopsy care and rehabilitation, which includes guidelines for rest, fluids, and following a prescribed diet. Comprehending the possible mental and physical obstacles that may arise during the recuperation stage enables people to manage the process more skillfully and enhance their general welfare.

CHAPTER TWO

THE ROLE OF NUTRITION IN HEALING

NUTRITION'S FUNCTION IN HEALING

To heal and recover from a variety of medical procedures and diseases, nutrition is essential. The body needs enough nutrients to support immune system activity, mend damaged tissues, and preserve general health; therefore the relationship between nutrition and recuperation is complex. For the body to mend itself more effectively and to maximize the healing process, a diet high in nutrients and well-balanced is necessary.

There are many different ways that nutrition affects recovery. Proteins, vitamins, minerals, and antioxidants are among the nutrients that are essential for encouraging tissue repair, lowering inflammation, and bolstering the body's defense systems. Particularly important for the healing process are proteins, which are needed for the synthesis of new tissues and the preservation of muscle mass. Sufficient consumption of protein promotes the synthesis of collagen and other structural proteins, which promote wound and surgical incision healing.

ADVANTAGES OF A DIET FOR PROSTATE BIOPSY RECOVERY

A recovery diet is crucial for certain medical operations, such as prostate biopsies, and its significance cannot be emphasized enough. One medical procedure that may induce pain and inflammation in the affected area is a prostate biopsy. A carefully thought-out recuperation diet might lessen these impacts and hasten the healing process. Consuming foods high in omega-3 fatty acids, fruits, and vegetables, which are anti-inflammatory, can help lessen the discomfort and inflammation brought on by the biopsy. Furthermore, it's critical to stay well hydrated throughout the healing process to promote overall body processes and eliminate toxins.

A prostate biopsy recovery diet has advantages that go beyond the short-term healing from the surgery.

A healthy diet can lower the chance of problems and promote long-term prostate health. Consuming foods high in antioxidants, such as green tea, tomatoes, and cruciferous vegetables, may protect prostate cells and lower the risk of oxidative stress and inflammation. Furthermore, as a healthy circulatory system is frequently associated with a lower risk of prostate problems, a diet that promotes overall cardiovascular health can also indirectly help prostate health.

THE NEED FOR NUTRITION DURING THE HEALING PROCESS

Customizing diet programs to meet the demands of each individual requires an understanding of the nutritional requirements during the healing process. Recovery may increase the body's energy expenditure, particularly if substantial tissue repair or surgery is required. To fulfill the increased energy demands, it is imperative to provide a sufficient calorie intake. Furthermore, to promote immune function and speed up the healing process, micronutrient requirements, such as those for vitamins and minerals, may be higher during recuperation.

It is impossible to exaggerate the role that diet plays in healing. During the healing process, a nutrient-dense, well-balanced diet is essential for fostering healing, lowering inflammation, and bolstering general health. Optimizing outcomes and encouraging long-term well-being requires customizing the diet to fit individual needs and taking into account the role of various nutrients, whether it's a general recuperation period or a specialized operation like a prostate biopsy.

CHAPTER THREE

CREATING A DIET PLAN FOR YOUR POST-BIOPSY RECOVERY

COLLABORATING WITH MEDICAL PROFESSIONALS

Creating a prostate biopsy recovery diet calls for careful planning, teamwork, and constant communication with medical specialists. Forming a solid alliance with medical professionals, such as urologists, nutritionists, and dietitians, is an essential first step. These experts are essential in comprehending the patient's particular medical condition and making recommendations that are tailored to meet their specific requirements and rehabilitation objectives.

When collaborating with medical specialists, a thorough evaluation of the patient's food choices, medical history, and current health issues is required. To make sure that the recovery diet supports healing and is in line with the overall treatment plan, open communication and dialogue are crucial. Medical practitioners can offer insightful information about the dietary needs that promote prostate biopsy healing, taking into consideration things like inflammation, possible adverse effects, and general health.

CUSTOMIZING A DIET TO EACH PERSON'S NEEDS

Creating a diet plan that is specific to each person's requirements is essential to creating a successful recovery strategy. Diets for prostate biopsy recuperation should be tailored to each patient's specific nutritional requirements and difficulties. To design a sustainable and pleasurable eating plan, individual differences in metabolism, dietary restrictions, and tastes must be taken into account.

By working closely with the patient, healthcare providers can better understand their goals, way of life, and cultural influences. This knowledge can be used to customize the diet so that it works well for the patient's everyday activities.

NUTRIENT ALIGNMENT FOR MAXIMUM RECUPERATION

One of the main ideas behind creating a prostate biopsy recovery diet is balancing nutrients for the best possible recovery. A varied range of nutrients, such as vitamins, minerals, proteins, carbs, and healthy fats, should be included in the diet. Sufficient consumption of protein is especially important for the immune system and tissue repair, which aid in the body's healing process. Fruits, vegetables, whole grains, and lean meats are nutrient-dense foods that should be given priority since they contain important vitamins and minerals that support general health.

Anti-inflammatory meals should also be included while balancing nutrients for the best possible recovery. A diet high in anti-inflammatory foods, such as fatty fish, nuts, seeds, and leafy greens, can help manage inflammation and promote healing.

Prostate biopsy treatments can cause inflammation. Staying hydrated is crucial for recuperation because it promotes healthy bodily functioning and facilitates the removal of pollutants.

Creating a prostate biopsy recovery diet requires working in tandem with medical specialists, who direct the procedure by recognizing each patient's unique demands. Customizing the diet to meet individual needs and tastes makes for a more long-lasting and successful healing strategy. A balanced diet that emphasizes anti-inflammatory foods helps support healing and general well-being while also supporting optimal recovery.

CHAPTER FOUR

ITEMS TO ADD TO YOUR DIET

FOODS THAT REDUCE INFLAMMATION

Including items that reduce inflammation in your diet is a smart move if you want to improve your general health and well-being. Numerous health problems, including rheumatoid arthritis, cardiovascular disease, and even some forms of cancer, have been related to chronic inflammation. Incorporating foods with anti-inflammatory qualities will help offset this. Omega-3 fatty acids, which are abundant in fatty fish like mackerel and salmon, have strong anti-inflammatory properties. Moreover, antioxidant-rich colorful fruits and vegetables like berries, cherries, and leafy greens help reduce inflammation at the cellular level.

RICH MINERAL AND VITAMIN SOURCES

To maintain maximum health, make sure your diet consists of a range of foods that are high in vitamins and minerals. These micronutrients are essential for several physiological functions, ranging from immune system support to bone health. Minerals like calcium and magnesium, as well as vitamins A, C, and K, are rich in leafy green vegetables like kale and spinach. Vitamin C, which is essential for collagen formation and immune system support, may be found in large amounts in citrus fruits like oranges and grapefruits. Including a variety of whole foods guarantees a balanced consumption of vital vitamins and minerals required for general health.

REHYDRATING TECHNIQUES FOR

Strategies for staying hydrated are essential for promoting healing and preserving general health. Maintaining proper hydration is essential for several body processes, such as nutrition transfer, temperature regulation, and digestion. The most important element of any hydration plan is water, so making sure you drink enough of it all day long is crucial. Eating foods high in water, such as cucumber, celery, and watermelon, can help maintain proper hydration levels.

Including foods and drinks high in electrolytes, such as bananas and coconut water, can also be very helpful in restoring electrolytes lost through perspiration, especially after vigorous exercise.

Promoting a healthy and balanced diet requires anti-inflammatory foods, a variety of vitamins and minerals, and efficient hydration techniques. These eating habits are important for long-term health promotion and recovery in addition to enhancing general well-being.

CHAPTER FIVE

FOODS NOT TO EAT WHILE RECOVERING

FOODS THAT MAY CAUSE INFLAMMATION AND BE IRRITANTS

It's critical to monitor the kinds of food you eat during the healing process since some meals can irritate the body and cause inflammatory reactions. Certain meals have the potential to worsen pre-existing medical issues, impede the healing process, and cause discomfort. Refined sugars, artificial additives, and highly processed foods are common irritants. Preservatives, colorings, and flavorings found in processed meals frequently have the potential to aggravate inflammation. Refined sugars, which are present in pastries, candies, and sugar-filled beverages, can also worsen the body's healing process and cause inflammation.

People in recovery should also avoid processed and sugar-filled foods, as well as foods high in trans and saturated fats.

Fried foods, quick food, and other processed snacks frequently include these bad fats. Diets heavy in fat have been linked to elevated inflammation, which could hinder the healing process. Focusing on a diet high in complete, unprocessed foods—such as fruits, vegetables, lean proteins, and whole grains—while reducing the consumption of certain irritants is advised to promote optimal recovery.

RESTRICTING SPECIFIC DRUGS TO PROMOTE BETTER HEALING

To encourage better healing results, people should think about restricting or abstaining from certain substances as they can impede the healing process. For example, drinking too much alcohol can weaken the immune system and interfere with the body's normal healing processes. Alcohol may also obstruct the body's ability to absorb vital nutrients, which would otherwise aid in the healing of tissues and organs. To maximize healing, it is recommended that those in recovery either abstain from alcohol entirely or use it sparingly.

Another drug that might need to be restricted when recovering is caffeine. While most people think that moderate amounts of caffeine are safe, excessive ingestion can cause dehydration and disrupt sleep cycles. The body needs both water and enough sleep to repair, and any disturbances in these areas might make it more difficult for the body to cure itself. It is advised to keep an eye on caffeine use and cut back if needed to promote general well-being while recovering.

RECOGNIZING FOODS THAT TRIGGER

People in recovery must understand trigger foods since they are particular foods that can worsen pre-existing medical disorders or cause unfavorable reactions. Foods that trigger different reactions in different people can vary based on personal allergies and sensitivities. Dairy products, grains containing gluten, shellfish, and some nuts are common trigger foods. Recognizing and avoiding trigger foods is essential for those recuperating from surgery, trauma, or disease to minimize difficulties and facilitate a quicker recovery.

Allergies and food sensitivities can present themselves as a variety of symptoms, including respiratory, skin, or digestive disorders. Maintaining a food journal or consulting with a medical practitioner can assist in identifying trigger foods and developing a customized eating plan that aids in the healing process. People can reduce their risk of inflammation, discomfort, and potential setbacks on their path to optimal health by being aware of and avoiding trigger foods.

CHAPTER SIX

EXAMPLE MENUS

OPTIONS FOR BREAKFAST

Eating a healthy, balanced breakfast first thing in the morning is crucial for giving the body the energy and nourishment it needs to speed up metabolism. Various breakfast options can accommodate varying nutritional needs and dietary preferences.

Options like Greek yogurt parfait with fruits and granola or scrambled eggs with veggies can be tasty and filling for individuals looking for a high-protein breakfast.

On the other hand, those who would rather have complex carbs could have porridge with nuts and berries or whole-grain toast with avocado. Incorporating a variety of macronutrients is essential for maintaining energy levels during the morning.

IDEAS FOR LUNCH

Lunch is a chance for midday fueling, and for maximum health and long-term vitality, it's important to include a variety of nutrients. A refreshing and satisfying choice can be a colorful salad with leafy greens, lean proteins like grilled chicken or tofu, and a variety of veggies. A filling and healthy lunch option is whole grain bowls or wraps with quinoa, beans, and roasted vegetables. Not only can adding healthy fats from avocados or olive oil improve flavor, but it also makes for a more filling and fulfilling dinner. Tailoring lunch selections to individual dietary requirements and taste preferences makes healthy eating more pleasurable and long-lasting.

RECIPES FOR DINNER

After a long day, dinner is a chance to relax and refuel with nutrition. A well-rounded dinner plate must have a variety of veggies, nutritious grains, and lean proteins. Appetizing and healthful dishes like stir-fried tofu, brown rice, and a rainbow of bright veggies, or grilled salmon with quinoa and steamed broccoli, can be prepared. Trying different combinations of herbs and spices can enhance flavor without sacrificing health. Including a range of veggies in the meal not only gives it vital vitamins and minerals but also gives it texture and visual attractiveness. Partition control and staying away from rich, thick sauces might help promote a more comfortable digestive process.

FOODS TO EAT FOR LONG-TERM ENERGY

Throughout the day, maintaining energy levels is mostly dependent on snacking. Choosing snacks that are high in protein and low in fiber can help control blood sugar levels and provide you with long-lasting energy.

Hummus and carrot sticks, nut and seed mixtures, and Greek yogurt with berries are all great options. Whole fruits, like bananas or apples, are light and portable snacks. A balanced snacking regimen can also benefit from including whole-grain options like rice cakes or whole-wheat crackers. For a snack to be both nutritious and pleasurable, it's important to pay attention to portion sizes and select foods that fit dietary requirements and personal tastes.

CHAPTER SEVEN

INCLUDING ADDENDA

SUMMARY OF SUGGESTED SUPPLEMENTS

A careful approach is needed when incorporating supplements into a daily routine, taking into account a variety of aspects such as dietary preferences, potential drug interactions, and individual health needs. A summary of suggested supplements might offer insightful information on the vital nutrients people should think about including to enhance their general health.

Minerals and vitamins are essential for good health, and while eating a balanced diet is the best way to get them, there are times when supplements are needed. For example, people with certain medical disorders, restricted diets, or those who have trouble getting enough nutrients from food alone may find it helpful to take supplements containing minerals like iron or vitamins like B12 or D.

But it's important to approach supplements with caution and realize that they shouldn't be used in place of a balanced diet.

WHEN AND HOW MUCH

Two important factors that affect the effectiveness of supplements are when and how much of them are taken. Knowing when and how to take supplements can have a big impact on how well the body absorbs and uses them. While some vitamins work best when taken with meals, some could be best taken on an empty stomach.

Supplement dosages should also be in line with personal needs and health objectives. Adhering to suggested guidelines is imperative to mitigate the risk of excessive consumption, which may result in unfavorable outcomes. Finding the right balance between excess and sufficiency is essential to getting the most out of supplements.

TALKING WITH MEDICAL PROFESSIONALS

Getting advice from medical professionals is an essential part of the supplementation procedure. Healthcare providers, including doctors, pharmacists, and registered dietitians, can offer individualized advice based on a patient's medical history, present conditions, and prescription regimen.

This consultation assists in pinpointing particular nutritional deficiencies and customizing supplement regimens to address them. In addition, medical professionals can provide valuable perspectives on any conflicts between prescription drugs and dietary supplements, guaranteeing that a person's general well-being is maintained.

It's critical to understand that everyone has different demands when it comes to supplements. Every person has different nutritional needs, which are influenced by a variety of factors including age, gender, lifestyle, and underlying medical conditions.

Therefore, it is not advisable to supplement in a way that is one size fits all. Instead, a thorough awareness of one's objectives and current state of health, along with expert guidance, serves as the foundation for an intelligent strategy for introducing supplements into a daily routine.

Adding supplements ought to be done so with awareness and a dedication to general well-being. A well-informed review of suggested supplements, cautious dosage and time planning, and consultation with medical professionals all add up to a plan that promotes personal health without sacrificing efficacy or safety.

CHAPTER EIGHT

LIFESTYLE FACTORS TO TAKE INTO ACCOUNT

THE VALUE OF EXERCISE

A healthy lifestyle is based on physical activity, which is essential for preserving general well-being. Participating in regular physical activity has numerous advantages, including better weight management, emotional modulation, and cardiovascular and muscle health.

Supporting a healthy body weight and lowering the risk factors linked to sedentary lifestyles, plays a crucial role in preventing chronic diseases like diabetes and heart disease. Beyond the obvious physical benefits, regular exercise promotes mental health by generating endorphins, which are the body's natural mood enhancers and help reduce stress and cultivate an optimistic outlook.

TECHNIQUES FOR STRESS MANAGEMENT

Stress has become a commonplace aspect of daily life in the fast-paced and demanding society we live in. Techniques for managing stress are essential for preserving emotional and mental balance. Deep breathing exercises and other mindfulness techniques can assist people in developing a sense of calmness and lessening the effects of stress. Since they lead to a more ordered and manageable daily schedule, time management techniques and goal-setting are also essential for stress management. Social support, from interpersonal connections to community involvement, also acts as a helpful stress reliever by promoting a feeling of community and shared experiences.

ADEQUATE REST AND SLEEP

Despite being essential building blocks of a healthy existence, adequate rest and sleep are sometimes disregarded in our hectic lives. Sleep is critical for both physical and mental healing, as it affects memory consolidation, cognitive processes, and emotional health in general. Prolonged sleep deprivation has been connected to several health problems, such as weakened immune systems, a higher chance of developing chronic illnesses, and mental health problems. Promoting optimal health requires establishing a regular sleep schedule, furnishing a cozy sleeping space, and placing a high priority on getting enough rest. Good sleep promotes a more balanced and satisfying existence by revitalizing the body and enhancing resilience to stress.

It is impossible to overestimate the significance of physical activity, stress reduction strategies, and enough rest and sleep within the framework of a balanced and healthful lifestyle. Incorporating these ideas into daily life fosters mental and emotional well-being in addition to physical health. People can develop a robust and balanced lifestyle that supports long-term health and happiness by making regular exercise a priority, implementing helpful stress management techniques, and realizing the importance of getting enough sleep.

CHAPTER NINE

KEEPING AN EYE ON AND MODIFYING YOUR DIET

FREQUENT CONSULTATIONS WITH MEDICAL EXPERTS

Consultations with medical professionals regularly are necessary for efficient diet monitoring and modification. These experts, which include physicians, nutritionists, and dietitians, are essential in offering individualized advice based on a person's health, medical background, and unique dietary requirements. Frequent consultations can aid in developing a thorough grasp of the person's general health as well as any conditions that may affect dietary decisions.

These check-ins make it easier to create a customized food plan that fits each person's health objectives. During these sessions, medical practitioners can evaluate variables like blood pressure, weight, cholesterol, and dietary deficits. By continuous observation, dietary modifications can be made to maximize nutritional intake in response to evolving situations or to address any new health issues.

IDENTIFYING SYMPTOMS OF CONCERN OR IMPROVEMENT

An essential part of keeping an eye on and modifying one's diet is recognizing indications of progress or concern. Positive indicators could indicate that the present nutritional plan is working, such as increased energy, improved mood, and consistent weight management. Conversely, warning indicators like inexplicable weight loss, ongoing exhaustion, or altered digestion ought to be closely monitored and promptly reported to medical experts.

Measuring mental and emotional health is part of tracking nutritional success in addition to physical signs. In addition to improving physical health, a balanced diet is crucial for maintaining mental and emotional equilibrium. Thus, it is essential for a thorough evaluation to identify any improvements or issues with mood, cognitive function, and general mental health.

Long-term dietary considerations include a comprehensive strategy for maintaining a long-term healthy lifestyle. While quick dietary adjustments could show effects right away, long-term success requires a realistic and consistent plan. Healthcare providers can help people form routines that are useful, pleasurable, and supportive of their general health.

Adapting to life transitions including aging, changes in physical activity, and changing health conditions is another important aspect of long-term dietary considerations. Patients can modify their diets in response to changing demands and circumstances by scheduling routine check-ins with healthcare specialists. Maintaining a healthy and balanced lifestyle and allowing for long-term changes in eating habits require flexibility.

Keeping an eye on your diet and making necessary adjustments calls for cooperation between patients and medical experts. Frequent check-ins offer insightful information about a person's health and enable tailored food plan modifications. Identifying indicators of progress or worry guarantees that favorable results are recognized and possible problems are quickly resolved. To enhance general health and well-being, long-term dietary concerns highlight the significance of sustainability, adaptation, and a holistic approach.

CHAPTER TEN

RECIPES FOR RECOVERING AFTER PROSTATE BIOPSY

SMOOTHIES PACKED WITH NUTRIENTS

Adding nutrient-packed smoothies to your diet can be a very healthy and tasty approach to fuel your body throughout the healing phase after a prostate biopsy. Smoothies are a quick and simple way to get the vital vitamins, minerals, and antioxidants needed for health and wellness in general. Try blending leafy greens like kale or spinach, which are high in vitamins and fiber, with a mixture of fruits, including berries that are high in antioxidants. Incorporating a source of protein, such as Greek yogurt or plant-based protein powder, can support both overall nutritional balance and muscle recovery. A dose of omega-3 fatty acids can be obtained by including chia or flaxseeds, which can have an anti-inflammatory impact. These nutrient-dense smoothies offer a delicious and refreshing method to stay hydrated in addition to aiding with healing.

SOUPS AND BROTHS THAT PROMOTE HEALING

Soups and broths that promote healing are an excellent way to replace key nutrients while providing a soothing and palatable choice for those recovering from a prostate biopsy. Go for soups with broth that are rich in whole grains, lean meats, and veggies. The nutrients in the soup support healing and strengthen the immune system, while the warmth of the dish can have a calming effect.

To further maximize the therapeutic advantages, add foods with anti-inflammatory qualities, such as ginger and garlic. Adding turmeric can also help reduce inflammation and promote general well-being because it contains the active component curcumin. For extra vitamins and a pleasing texture, try adding root veggies like sweet potatoes and carrots. These therapeutic soups are a wholesome and nutritious complement to the diet during recuperation.

HEALTHY MAIN COURSES

It's critical to concentrate on consuming filling main courses that offer a well-balanced combination of proteins, healthy fats, and carbohydrates when you recuperate after your prostate biopsy. Since protein is necessary for tissue regeneration and recovery, choose lean protein sources such as grilled chicken, fish, or tofu. Include nutritious grains, such as brown rice or quinoa, which give complex carbohydrates and a slow-burning energy source.

When it comes to bolstering the immune system, vegetables—especially those high in vitamins A and C—should take center stage in your main courses. To add healthy fats, aid in nutrition absorption, and support heart health, try drizzling olive oil or adding avocado. T

he secret is to prepare tasty and nutrient-dense meals that will provide your body with the building blocks it needs to heal quickly.

DESSERTS AND SNACKS

You can still enjoy and vary your diet with desserts and snacks while recovering after a prostate biopsy by sticking to a nutrient-dense diet. Choose more nutritious dessert options instead of sugary ones, like fruit salads, yogurt parfaits, or dark chocolate with almonds. These will still fulfill your sweet needs while providing essential nutrients. A balanced intake of vitamins and healthy fats can be obtained from snacks, so choose wisely. Nuts, seeds, and dried fruits are good choices. Think about including anti-inflammatory snacks, such as a handful of walnuts or almonds, which are high in omega-3 fatty acids. When choosing snacks and desserts, moderation is essential to make sure they enhance total nutrient intake and help you heal from a prostate biopsy.

www.ingramcontent.com/pod-product-compliance
Lightning Source LLC
Chambersburg PA
CBHW060814260726
48660CB00002B/952